Usually when ordering a chocolate dessert

I remember the last time I ever did it.

I was having dinner with a new acquaintance and he didn't even crack a smile when I made light of the heavy meal I had put away.

He looked me up and down and revealed that he, too, used to be 30 pounds overweight with a ready stock of silly excuses when faced with a menu.

"Like you, I didn't exercise and looked like a statistic waiting to happen", he said. "So when my heart attack arrived, a year ago today, I could hardly pretend that it came out of a clear blue sky.

"The stupid thing is," he went on, "I'd known exactly how to avoid it. Do a bit more, eat a bit less, cut down the salt and the alcohol. The advice isn't hidden away, is it? Nor is it complicated."

"So why didn't you do something?" I asked.

And his reply stopped me short.

I'LL JUST HAVE A SKINNY LATTE, THANKS

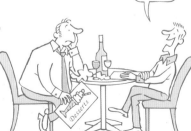

3

I WASN'T SCARED ENOUGH

He said he didn't know that sudden death creeps up on you

He thought there was plenty of time to lose weight and start exercising.

"I'm not that old!" He'd say. "I'm in the prime of life! I still have wild oats to sow (or at least, wild mushroom omelettes to enjoy)."

There was nothing and no-one staring him in the face and saying *Do it now or else.*

"Or, rather," he said, "there wasn't until a year ago. A year ago, I woke up in hospital, festooned with wires and drips, surrounded by a worried family, to receive a resounding lecture from a large, fierce doctor.

"She congratulated me on surviving my first heart attack and said the next one would get me for sure.

"My only chance was to lose weight, get fit and stop taking breathing for granted."

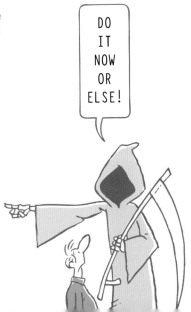

NOW, YOU CAN BE AS LUCKY AS MY FRIEND

Yes, he was glad he'd had a heart attack

He didn't think so at the time, of course. But in the 12 months afterwards, he realised it was the kick in the pants he needed to give himself a longer life.

He got scared enough to lose weight.

Frightened enough to get fitter.

Worried enough to walk the dog instead of watching tv all evening.

Terrified enough to tackle his drinking, his salt, his cream puffs and his pies.

"Barring unforeseen encounters with a bus," he said to me that night, "there's now a good chance I can look forward to more happy, healthy years than I could have done *before* I was rushed to hospital! In short, my heart attack has helped me to live longer."

He certainly looked better than I did, so I asked him to explain how he had done it, step by step. And I also got permission to share his system with you, on condition that I didn't change a word.

So here it is, exactly as told to me.

7

FIRST, LET ME TELL YOU WHAT I DIDN'T DO

I didn't join a gym

There's nothing wrong with working out, but I've joined a gym twice before and never kept it up for longer than a month or so. Instead, I built more activity into the things I do already.

I didn't go on a diet

They're great, until you stop, and then you put the weight back on. Why? I think it's because we see them as a temporary fix, when what we need is a permanent change in the way we eat.

I didn't rush

I was so scared at first, I would have signed up for any crash diet and workout plan on offer. But at the same time, I didn't know how my heart would cope with exertion.

So instead, I chose to do things steadily, losing a pound or two a month and exercising little and often, rather than to the point of exhaustion.

So. Would you like to hear my plan?

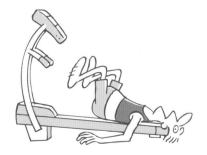

STEP 1

I took more steps

In a typical day, I realised that sitting down was my favourite position and activity was unusual. I decided to change the ratio around.

STEP 2

I ate more food

But I ate food that was better for me and I ate it the right way - regularly, slowly, socially.

STEP 3

I took control

This wasn't some
half-hearted pipe-dream,
it was life or death,
so I used some simple
thinking and planning
techniques to make sure
I stayed the course.

Ready for
step 1?

STEP 1, TAKE MORE STEPS

Don't sit still for more than 10 minutes

If you spend most of your time at rest at the moment (sitting, lying, standing still) this needs to stop right now.

If you sit at a desk or in front of the TV a lot, get hold of a cooking timer and set it to remind you to get up and walk around every 10 minutes. Walk for 1 minute. If there are some stairs handy, go up and down these a couple of times.

If you're not allowed to leave your desk so often, use your breaks and lunchtime to take a short walk or walk up and down stairs.

If you're in an active job already, or on your feet in a shop, perhaps, you need to work up more of a sweat. Use the stairs again or, if you can, do what you already do but do it faster, 'till you're out of breath.

So that's the little walks. Now for the big ones.

WALK TWICE A WEEK FOR AN HOUR

You'll lose worries as well as weight

Phone a good friend and say 'Congratulations! You're on the keeping me alive team!'

Arrange to meet at least twice a week and take a 60-minute walk together.

Try and walk somewhere hilly, or pretty, or interesting. Or change your route regularly so there's variety and always something to talk about.

If you have hills in your walk, don't slow down for them, try and keep the same pace as on the flat. If you don't have hills, try to walk fast so that you get out of breath.

And while you're walking, really notice what's around you.
The wind, the warmth, the cold, the trees, the flowers, the shops and the sky

After a few weeks you'll notice two things - A, you're a bit fitter and B, you're a bit happier.

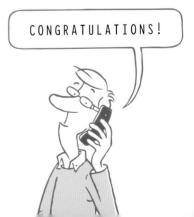

CONGRATULATIONS!

NOW CHANGE THE WAY YOU SHOP AND TRAVEL

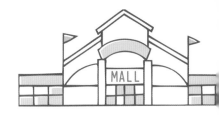

A shopping mall can make you thin

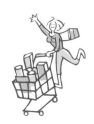

Shopping centres, car parks, bus stops – they're all great for exercise.

When you're parking at the supermarket, choose a space that's long way from the entrance and walk briskly to the door.

In the mall, take the stairs, not the escalator or elevator. On bus rides, get off a stop early so you have to walk a bit further to your destination.

Think about your regular journeys and choose to walk the ones that are less than a mile. Yes, you may need to take an umbrella sometimes! Yes, you might need an overcoat or waterproof jacket! No, you can't do this bit on sunny days only!

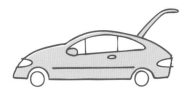

HEAVY BREATHIN KEEPS YOU BREATHIN

Improve the exercise you do already.

Household chores are exercise. So is washing the car and gardening. When you lift or move things at work or school, that's exercise too.

So why aren't you slim and lovely? Because you're not doing it fast enough.

Exercise only works properly when you get out of breath and your heart starts pumping.

So do the housework faster. Clean the car quicker. Move those files or shift those boxes at a run. Fit some brisk cardio-vascular exercise into your day (always being careful not to take risks or hurt yourself of course).

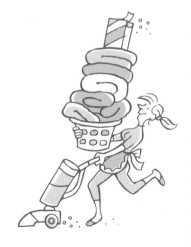

GET DISORGANISED – IT'S GOOD FOR YOU

Have you noticed? Headless chickens are seldom overweight

If you have one of those boxes at the bottom of the stairs that collect things so that you can make fewer trips up and down, move it to the attic, you don't need it any more.

If you're the sort that's really organised in the kitchen or at work – saving wasted motion and unnecessary walking about - stop it, now.

Wasted motion is good. Going upstairs dozens of times a day is great. Making three trips to the stationery cupboard is better than carrying three things in one trip.

Activity – any activity- keeps you alive. Sitting down doesn't.

And that's step 1 of my plan. Now get up, walk up and down the stairs twice, and turn the page for step 2.

STEP 2, EAT MORE FOOD

Whatever you do, don't go on a diet

You'll only get fat again when you come off it.

A diet is like any short-term fix – short term. I'm interested in long-term solutions here, so don't bother with the books or the magazine articles, the carbs, the calorie counting or the combining.

Don't get me wrong, they all work if you need to shrink an inch or so in time for the holidays. But if you want more time on planet earth, you need another approach entirely.

What you do is eat *more*, not *less*, using and enjoying different foods in a natural way, so that you lose excess fat gently and permanently, while feeling and looking better at the same time.

You'll also feel more energetic, which is just as well with all that walking I had you doing in step 1.

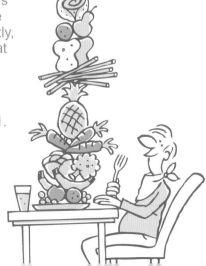

HOW YOU EAT

...is almost as important as what you eat

Have you noticed that in cultures with great food, fewer people are fat?

That's because they love to eat. They prepare their food carefully. They treat mealtimes as a big deal. They love sitting down with family and friends. And they linger over every mouthful because it tastes so good.

So make yourself these promises, right now:

• I promise to stop and have a meal, three times a day, at roughly the same time each day

• I promise not to eat standing up, at the fridge, in the car or on the run

• I promise to switch off the TV while eating a meal

• I promise to prepare my own food from fresh ingredients as often as I can

• I promise to eat with other people as often as possible

You're too busy to change your relationship with food? You can't possibly stop and eat a proper meal that often? Preparing fresh food just doesn't fit your lifestyle?

Fair enough. It's your funeral.

NOW HERE'S WHAT TO EAT

There's so much advice on this, I didn't know where to turn or who to believe at first. But then I hit on the idea of finding someone that doesn't have a book to sell or a food range to promote and is required, by law, to give advice that's based on scientific evidence.

That someone is called N.I.C.E. – the National Institute for Health and Clinical Excellence – and it seemed to me that ignoring their advice would be a bit like saying "Shut up and get me chocolate." to the big, fierce doctor in the cardiac ward.

and I quote . . .

Base your meals on starchy foods such as potatoes, bread, rice and pasta, choosing wholegrain where possible.

Eat plenty of fibre-rich foods such as oats, beans, peas, lentils, grains, seeds, fruit and vegetables, as well as wholegrain bread, and brown rice and pasta.

Eat at least five portions of fruit and vegetables a day in place of foods higher in fat and calories.

Choose low-fat foods.

Avoid foods containing a lot of fat and sugar, such as fried food, sweetened drinks, sweets and chocolate.

Avoid taking in too many calories in the form of alcohol.

I know. It's a bit boring isn't it? So there's something to cheer you up over the page.

ONE TREAT A DAY IS OK

But when the menu says 'Death by Chocolate' it means it

Sorry, but you'll have to forget about big desserts, especially at the end of a meal when you're already full.

But there's nothing wrong with a little treat every day, so long as you have just one.

Some people set aside a time in the evening for a square of chocolate or a biscuit. Others treat themselves to a bag of chips at lunchtime. Others just love a nice lump of cheese, so they have one, every day.

So long as treats are just that, and most of your eating takes place at mealtimes, you'll be fine.

Of course, you could always train yourself to nibble fruit or vegetables between meals. If you can do this you are, of course, rather strange, but it does mean you can have as many treats as you like.

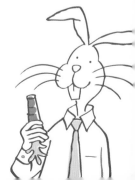

GOOD NEWS!

BREAKFAST
MAKES YOU
SMALLER

The first of your 3 meals a day is the most important

You really can eat more and weigh less, especially if you do most of your eating at breakfast time. What's that? You can't face breakfast? That's what I used to say BHA (before heart attack).

Trouble is, when you do without breakfast, your body doesn't get the right kind of start and it sulks all day, demanding snacks and often giving you a headache by lunchtime.

But if you have porridge, muesli or bran cereal each morning, you'll feel full until lunch. You won't want to nibble and your digestion will be working away, using up calories, which makes you thinner.

There's something else I should mention, if you don't mind. Porridge and muesli work like – how can I put this – drain unblockers. After a few days they clear your system out and you feel better all round.

WHEN YOU CAN'T FACE ANOTHER MANGO

An easy way to get your 5 a day

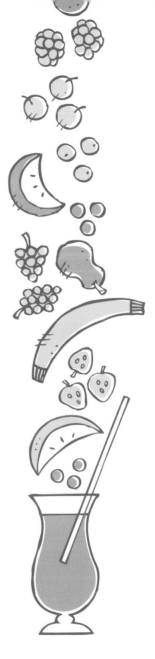

Even if you like fruit and vegetables, it's sometimes hard to have five portions of it every day.

Trouble is, you really do need that much fibre. Without it, your system clogs up and you get all sad and sluggish as well as short-lived and fat.

So here's a cheat – drink smoothies.

All you need is a blender (liquidisers and food processors work as well) and some fruit. Fresh is good, but frozen is fine, too, especially in summer.

There's no right or wrong way to make a smoothie – use your favourite fruits and make it as thick or as runny as you like. Some people even make their smoothies not very smooth, with chunks of fruit to chew on. These are called lumpies.

NOW, ABOUT THE BOOZE

A glass of wine is like a chocolate bar

It's all very well NICE saying *avoid taking in too many calories in the form of alcohol* but how many is too many and how do you get down to the right amount?

This was one of the things I struggled with, so I had to develop some plans and little routines that kept me on the straight and narrow.

You'll find them in step 3, but another thing that worked for me was comparing the bad news in drinks to other stuff.

For example, if you like a beer did you know that, calorifically speaking, every pint is the same as a Cadbury's Creme Egg?

You wouldn't eat 4 Kit Kats a night, would you? But I used to have 4 glasses of wine occasionally, and both options amount to almost 500 calories!

I'd remind myself of this each evening if I weakened. It stopped me sidling up to the wine rack for another bottle of Shiraz.

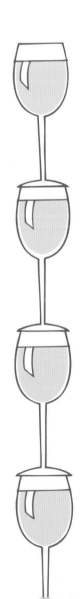

YOU DON'T NEED BATHROOM SCALES

Your tummy will tell you how you're doing

Forget about kilos, pounds and ounces. In the same way that the waistband on your skirt or trousers has been your early warning system for years (even though you've been ignoring it), it is now your bringer of glad tidings.

So long as you're losing that tightness around the middle, and maybe even trying on stuff you used to be able to get into years ago, you're fine.

There's another reason your waist is important. The bigger it is, the more likely you are to develop health problems.

If you're a man, over 94cm (37 inches) is the danger zone. You need to do something about it. Over 102 cm (40 inches) and it's urgent.

If you're a woman, 80cm (32 inches) is the red line and the alarm really goes off at 88cm (35 inches).

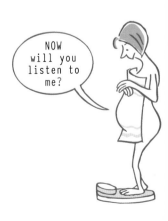

NOW will you listen to me?

DON'T BE A ROLY-POLY ROLE MODEL

When you eat better, your kids do, too

If you have kids, you'll want to help them avoid a heart attack in later life. So sit down at a table and eat with them. All eat the same thing, by the way - they can't have pizza or burgers while you're having pasta.

Now tell them that this is how it's going to be from now on. Like it or not, the family is going to be together for at least five meals a week, chewing, chatting and generally behaving like a TV commercial.

After a while, they'll get into the same good food habits as you, staying healthier throughout their lives and never having to buy books like this.

You might also try inviting them on your long walks, and before you reply "You wouldn't say that if you knew my kids", bear in mind that emotional blackmail can be quite effective.

"So you're refusing to help me avoid a heart attack, then?"

STEP 3, TAKE CONTROL

You decide whether this will work or not

The heart attack, if you have it, will be yours and yours alone, so let's get something straight - success or failure is entirely in your hands. Correction: in your mind.

So I've gathered some tips and techniques that will help you deal with the doubts and difficulties you will face.

I'll help you:

Renew the resolve. Even though I was scared, I couldn't maintain my enthusiasm every minute. I needed reminders and reasons to keep going.

Cope with cravings. There were times when I was desperate for a snack. Other times I was so bored with eating properly that I just had to get a doughnut!

See off self-doubt. Can I really do this? Am I strong enough to reduce my drinking? Maybe I don't have the will power to cut out chips?

Dump depression. Once or twice I got really fed up. Life felt flat, and it seemed that my only options were death or broccoli!

Set up a support network. I really wished that I knew someone who had also a heart attack, and we were doing this together.

WHAT (OR WHO) ARE YOUR REASONS TO LIVE?

Write them down and keep them in your pocket

You've got to see your children graduate. Then there are the weddings. And the grandkids. And the Nobel Prizes. Or maybe you need to make it past 100!

So stick their pictures in a little album and keep it in your wallet or purse, for those moments of weakness.

Other reasons? Then pepper your fridge with post-it notes.

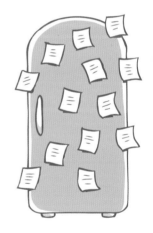

Write messages on them about why you want to live longer, what it will be like when you're slimmer and fitter and how great you're going to feel in the extra years you're giving to yourself.

Stick notes everywhere you'll see them and then, once a week, move them around so you don't get so used to them that you take no notice.

DON'T JUST SIT THERE, MAKE A PLAN!

Make this a project, not a daydream

Decide what you're going to do, and work out how you'll do it.

Write your plan down, step by step. Be sure to make them small, simple steps that you will be able to do.

Keep a diary of how the plan is going. Check progress and if things aren't going well, work out how to get back on track.

Remember, you're working on living longer – there can't be anything more important than that!

Turn over for tips on how to plan

THINK
ABOUT
ELEPHANTS

You can do anything if you break it into bits

How do you eat an elephant?
In lots of little mouthfuls.

It's the same with changes to your eating and exercise patterns.
Even if your task looks enormous, you *will* be able to do it if you break it into bits.

Let's say you want to cut down drinking. You could start by breaking the week into pieces and just stop on Mondays, for example.

It's the same with your weight. Don't stare at the whole elephant and say "Oh no! I have to lose 20 pounds!", break the task up into 1 pound chunks and work on them one at a time.

Most objectives can be chopped up like this, and you're much more likely to succeed when you do things bit by bit.

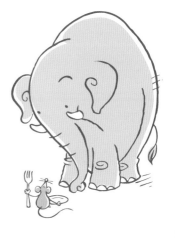

WHAT
IF
YOU
GET
STUCK?

Don't worry, everyone does

Everybody gets discouraged. Nobody can sail straight through an important change in life like this without feeling fed up or going off the rails sometimes.

There are two things you must do about this:

1. Expect to get stuck from time to time

2. Work out what to do about it *in advance*

There are lots of things that can help you through the bad patches.

Check the next few pages for ideas.

GET YOUR FRIENDS AND FAMILY ON THE TEAM

Don't try and do this alone

The more people you involve in your project, the more likely it is to work out.

Right from the start, tell all the people you trust what you're doing and ask for their support.

They'll be there for you when you slip, or when doubts set in. Call them up and tell them how you feel.

If you have someone very close – a partner, husband, wife, best friend - ask him or her to be your conscience.

When you get stuck, he or she will remind you why you're doing this and may even tell you things you don't want to hear!

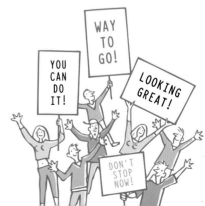

GIVE YOURSELF SOME GOOD ADVICE

What would you say to your best friend?

If you're feeling really stuck, this often works:

Imagine it's not you who's trying to get slimmer and healthier, but your best friend. He or she was doing really well but has now slipped a little.

What would you say? How would you remind your friend that all those extra years will be great? How would you gently encourage him or her to get back on track?

Now say all that to yourself. Give yourself the advice and support that you'd give to your very best friend. You deserve it.

SIT RIGHT DOWN AND WRITE YOURSELF A LETTER

Do it now, while you're all fired up

Imagine it's ten years from now and you're sitting down to write a thank you letter to yourself.

Life is great - so much better than it used to be - and you want to thank the person you were ten years ago for persevering, making the changes and creating such a great, long term future.

What would you write? Get a pen and paper and start that letter now. It might begin like this:

Hi!

I want to say thanks for persevering all those years ago. Without your efforts and determination, I probably wouldn't be here…

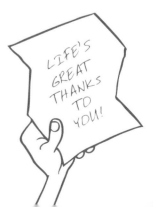

KNOW HOW TO BEAT THOSE NIBBLE CRAVINGS

They only last 5 minutes

I know how it feels to *need* a snack. You can't think of anything but that bag of chips or chocolate bar.

As it happens, cravings like this are manufactured by your mind and only last about 5 minutes! To beat them, all you have to do is get through the 5-minute spells, one by one, until they go away for good.

So next time you feel a craving coming on, follow the plan over the page and I promise you'll win the battle of wills with yourself!

1. Say Hello.

When you notice a nibble-craving coming on, mentally step back, see it for what it is, and let it know.

"Hello craving. You're trying to make me nibble, but you can't. And you'll be dead in 5 minutes!"

When you treat a craving this way, it loses most of its power over you. By knowing it's there, naming it and remembering that it won't last long, you've taken control of the situation.

2. Say Goodbye.

Now speak to the craving again, saying "Not today, thank you!" and turn your back on it.

Don't challenge it or try to argue with it, don't think about it any more, just let it be. A craving loves attention, so don't give it any.

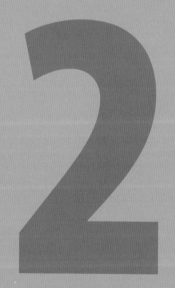

3. Do Your Thing.

Having spotted the nibble craving for what it is and sent it away to a corner, you may now use its short and miserable life to enhance your own.

Yes, you have 5 minutes free time in which to do anything you like. You used to spend it eating flapjacks or Danish pastries, but now you can spend it on yourself. I call it Doing Your Thing.

You might do a 5-minute meditation. Look through family photos to remember why you want to live longer.

You might recite a favourite poem to yourself, or memorise a new one.

You could read part of a book, play music, do press-ups with a friend, learn to draw, write a letter, touch your toes, do a crossword or sudoku.

There are just 2 rules – Your Thing must last about 5 minutes (like a craving), and it must be enjoyable or useful (unlike a craving).

DON'T HIDE INSIDE COVER-UP CLOTHING

Buy those smaller sizes now

If you've taken to wearing extra roomy clothes that hide your shape, it's time to take them to the second-hand shop.

Hiding your figure was the same as hiding from the truth and you're not going to do that any more. In fact you're going to do the opposite.

Buy some stuff that will fit in six months, but is too tight now, and wear it every day.

The tightness will be uncomfortable, but it will remind you of your goal and of those dangerous waist measurements. It'll also help stop you nibbling.

What's more, you'll really feel the benefit when you start to lose inches around your middle!

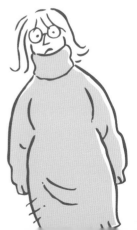

YOU'RE ONLY 3 STEPS AWAY FROM A LONGER LIFE

STEP 1. Take more steps

Give your bum a break by never sitting on it for more than 10 minutes at a time. Get up, walk around, climb stairs, work up a sweat, be inefficient, use the mall as an exercise opportunity, get off the bus early, walk with a friend, don't drive less than a mile and never, ever park near the entrance to anywhere.

STEP 2. Eat more food

So long as it's high fibre, low fat and so delicious you want to linger over every mouthful. Have breakfast, make smoothies, prepare meals, sit down with friends and kids, switch off the TV, don't diet, watch your waist and think of every glass of wine as a bar of chocolate.

STEP 3. Take control

Make the album, write the reasons, cover the fridge, make the plan, eat the elephant, do your thing, phone a friend, write the letter, donate the clothes and remember, only one person gets to decide whether you succeed or fail, and you're it!

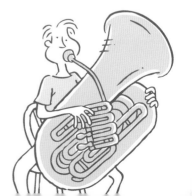

SO:

YOU'LL BE HAPPIER

YOU'LL BE FITTER

YOU'LL LOOK BETTER

AND YOU'LL LIVE LONGER

You better have a really good reason for not starting right this minute!

I,..

Do solemnly promise that I will make a plan to live longer by taking more steps, eating more food and taking control, starting on

....

GOOD LUCK!

HELP WITH
OTHER
THINGS
IN YOUR
LIFE

This little book is one of a series by Dr Chris Williams that offer real, practical solutions to most of the things life throws at us.

The full range is shown opposite and they're all available at **www.fiveareas.com** or from many healthcare practitioners.

There's also a free web site, **www.livinglifetothefull.com** where you can get advice, deal with problems and connect with other people who are using food and exercise to give themselves the chance of a longer life.